The Complete Keto

Recipe Book 2021

The Ultimate Keto Diet Recipe Book

The Healthy Way to Lose Weight

and Improve Mood

Tanya Scofield

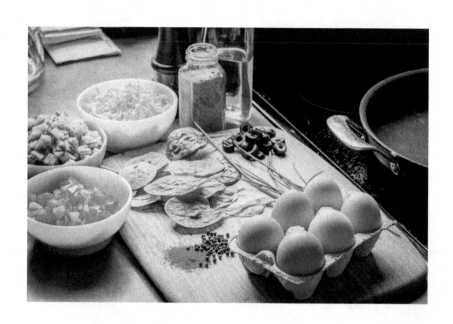

Table of Contents

consent from the Publisher. All additional right reserved.

The information in the following pages is broadly considered a truthful and accurate account of facts and as such, any inattention, use, or misuse of the information in question by the reader will render any resulting actions solely under their purview. There are no scenarios in which the publisher or the original author of this work can be in any fashion deemed liable for any hardship or damages that may befall them after undertaking information described herein.

Additionally, the information in the following pages is intended only for informational purposes and should thus be thought of as universal. As befitting its nature, it is presented without assurance regarding its prolonged validity or interim quality. Trademarks that are mentioned are done without written consent and can in no way be considered an endorsement from the trademark holder.

INTRODUCTION

So the Ketogenic Diet is all about reducing the amount of carbohydrates you eat. Does this mean you won't get the kind of energy you need for the day? Of course not! It only means that now, your body has to find other possible sources of energy. Do you know where they will be getting that energy? Even before we talk about how to do keto – it's important to first consider why this particular diet works. What actually happens to your body to make you lose weight? As you probably know, the body uses food as an energy source. Everything you eat is turned into energy, so that you can get up and do whatever you need to accomplish for the day. The main energy source is sugar so what happens is that you eat something, the body breaks it down into sugar, and the sugar is processed into energy. Typically, the "sugar" is taken directly from the food you eat so if you eat just the right amount of food, then your body is fueled for the whole day. If you eat too much, then the sugar is stored in your body – hence the accumulation of fat.

But what happens if you eat less food? This is where the Ketogenic Diet comes in. You see, the process of creating sugar from food is usually faster if the food happens to be rich in carbohydrates. Bread, rice, grain, pasta – all of these are carbohydrates and they're the easiest food types to turn into energy.

So here's the situation – you are eating less carbohydrates every day. To keep you energetic, the body breaks down the stored fat and turns them into molecules called ketone bodies. The process of turning the fat into ketone bodies is called "Ketosis" and obviously – this is where the name of the Ketogenic Diet comes from. The ketone bodies take the place of glucose in keeping you energetic. As long as you keep your carbohydrates reduced, the body will keep getting its energy from your body fat.

The Ketogenic Diet is often praised for its simplicity and when you look at it properly, the process is really straightforward. The Science behind the effectivity of the diet is also well-documented, and has been proven multiple times by different medical fields. For example, an article on Diet Review by Harvard provided a lengthy discussion on how the Ketogenic Diet works and why it is so effective for those who choose to use this diet.

But Fat Is the Enemy...Or Is It?

No – fat is NOT the enemy. Unfortunately, years of bad science told us that fat is something you have to avoid – but it's actually a very helpful thing for weight loss! Even before we move forward with this book, we'll have to discuss exactly what "healthy fats" are, and why they're actually the good guys. To do this, we need to make a distinction between the different kinds of fat. You've probably heard of them before and it is a little bit confusing at first. We'll try to go through them as simply as possible:

Saturated fat. This is the kind you want to avoid. They're also called "solid fat" because each molecule is packed with hydrogen atoms. Simply put, it's the kind of fat that can easily cause a blockage in your body. It can raise cholesterol levels and lead to heart problems or a stroke. Saturated fat is something you can find in meat, dairy products, and other processed food items. Now, you're probably wondering: isn't the Ketogenic Diet packed with saturated fat? The answer is: not necessarily. You'll find later in the recipes given that the Ketogenic Diet promotes primarily unsaturated fat or healthy fat. While there are definitely many meat recipes in the list, most of these recipes contain healthy fat sources.

Unsaturated Fat. These are the ones dubbed as healthy fat. They're the kind of fat you find in avocado, nuts, and other ingredients you usually find in Keto-friendly recipes. They're known to lower blood cholesterol and actually come in two types: polyunsaturated and monounsaturated. Both are good for your body but the benefits slightly vary, depending on what you're consuming.

Dill Bell Pepper Bowls

Preparation Time: 10 minutes

Cooking Time: 0 minutes

Servings: 4

Ingredients:

- 2 tablespoons dill, chopped
- 1 yellow onion, chopped
- 1 pound multi colored bell peppers, cut into halves, seeded and cut into thin strips
- 3 tablespoons olive oil
- 2 and ½ tablespoons white vinegar
- Black pepper to the taste

Directions:

1. In a salad bowl, mix bell peppers with onion, dill, pepper, oil and vinegar, toss to coat, divide into small bowls and serve as a snack.

Nutrition: Calories 120 Fat 3 Fiber 4 Carbs 2 Protein 3

Baked Lemon & Pepper Chicken

Preparation Time: 20 minutes

Cooking Time: 25 minutes

Servings: 4

Ingredients:

- 4 chicken breast fillets
- Salt to taste
- 1 tablespoon olive oil
- 1 lemon, sliced thinly
- 1 tablespoon maple syrup
- 2 tablespoons lemon juice
- 2 tablespoons butter
- Pepper to taste

Directions:

1. Preheat your oven to 425 degrees F.
2. Season chicken with salt.
3. Pour oil into a pan over medium heat.
4. Cook chicken for 5 minutes per side.
5. Transfer chicken to a baking pan.
6. Surround the chicken with the lemon slices.
7. Bake in the oven for 10 minutes.
8. Pour in maple syrup and lemon juice to the pan.
9. Put the butter on top of the chicken.

10.Sprinkle with pepper.

11.Bake for another 5 minutes.

Nutrition: Calories 286 Total Fat 13 g Saturated Fat 5 g Cholesterol 109 mg Sodium 448 mg Total Carbohydrate 7 g Dietary Fiber 1.4 g Protein 34.8 gTotal Sugars 3 g Potassium 350 mg

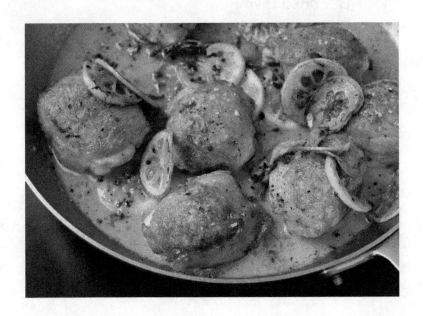

Skillet Chicken with White Wine Sauce

Preparation Time: 5 minutes

Cooking Time: 30 minutes

Servings: 4

Ingredients:

- 4 boneless chicken thighs
- 1 tsp. garlic powder
- 1 tsp. dried thyme
- 1 tbsp. olive oil
- 1 tbsp. butter
- 1 yellow onion diced
- 3 garlic cloves minced
- 1 cup dry white wine
- ½ cup heavy cream
- fresh chopped parsley
- salt and pepper

Directions:

1. Heat your oil in a skillet. Season your chicken, add it to the skillet, and then cook it about 5-7 mins.
2. Flip the chicken and cook until looking golden brown.

3. Remove the chicken to a plate.

4. Add butter to the skillet. Then add onions and cook them until softened.

5. Stir in garlic salt and pepper, add wine and cook for 4-5 mins.

6. Stir in the thyme and the heavy cream.

7. Place the breasts back to the skillet and leave to simmer for 2-3 mins. Top them with the parsley.

Nutrition: Calories: 276 kcal Fats: 21 g Carbs: 6 g Protein: 25 g

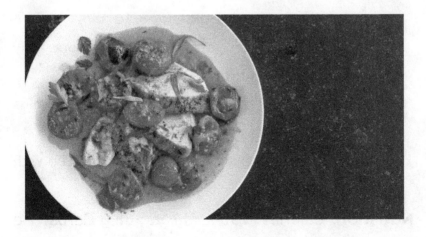

Stir Fry Kimchi and Pork Belly

Preparation Time: 10 minutes

Cooking Time: 18 minutes

Servings: 3

Ingredients:

- 300 g pork belly
- 1 lb. kimchi
- 1 tbsp. soy sauce
- 1 tbsp. rice wine
- 1 tbsp. sesame seeds
- 1 stalk green onion

Directions:

1. Slice the pork as thin as possible and marinate it in soy sauce and rice wine for 8-10 mins.
2. Heat a pan. When very hot, add the pork belly and stir-fry until brown.
3. Add the kimchi to the pan and stir-fry for 2 mins to let the flavors completely mix.
4. Turn off heat and slice the green onion. Top with sesame seeds.

Nutrition: Calories: 790 kcal Fats: 68 g Carbs: 7 g Protein: 14 g

Lemon Butter Sauce with Fish

Preparation Time: 10 minutes

Cooking Time: 10 minutes

Servings: 2

Ingredients:

- 150 g thin white fish fillets
- 4 tbsps. butter
- 2 tbsps. white flour
- 2 tbsps. olive oil
- 1 tbsp. fresh lemon juice
- salt and pepper
- chopped parsley

Directions:

1. Place the butter in a small skillet over medium heat. Melt it and leave it, just stirring it casually. After 3 mins, pour into a small bowl.
2. Add lemon juice and season it and set it aside.
3. Dry the fish with paper towels, season it to taste, and sprinkle with flour.
4. Heat oil in a skillet over high heat: when shimmering, add the fish and cook around 2-3 mins.

5. Remove to a plate and serve with the sauce. Top with parsley.

Nutrition: Calories: 371 kcal Fats: 27 g Carbs: 3 g Protein: 30 g

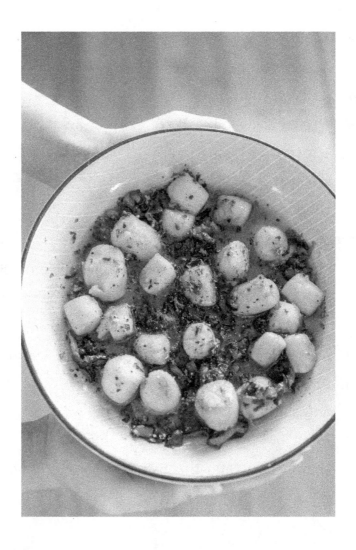

Pressure Cooker Crack Chicken

Preparation Time: 5 minutes

Cooking Time: 25 minutes

Servings: 8

Ingredients:

- 2 lbs. boneless chicken thighs.
- 2 slices bacon
- 8 ozs. cream cheese
- 1 scallion sliced
- ½ cup shredded cheddar
- 1 ½ tsp. garlic and onion powder
- 1 tsp. red pepper flakes and dried dill
- salt and pepper
- 2 tbsps. apple cider vinegar
- 1 tbsp. dried chives

Directions:

1. On pressure cooker, use sauté mode and wait for it to heat up. Add the bacon and cook until crispy. Then set aside on a plate.
2. Add everything in the pot, except the cheddar cheese. On Manual high, pressure cook them for 15 mins and then release it.

3. On a large plate, shred the chicken and then return to the pot and the cheddar.

4. Top with the bacon and scallion.

Nutrition: Calories: 437 kcal Fats: 28 g Carbs: 5 g Protein: 41 g

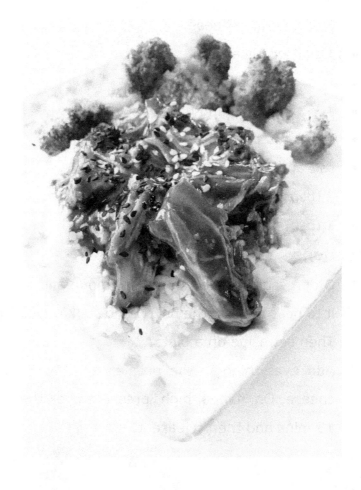

Bacon Bleu Cheese Filled Eggs

Preparation Time: 10 minutes

Cooking Time: 90-120 minutes

Servings: 3

Ingredients:

- 8 eggs
- ¼ cup crumbled bleu cheese
- 3 slices of cooked bacon
- ¼ cup sour cream
- 1/3 cup mayo
- ¼ tsp. pepper and dill
- ½ tsp. salt
- 1 tbsp. mustard
- parsley

Directions:

1. Hard boil your eggs and then cut them half. Place the yolks in a bowl.
2. With a fork, mash the yolks, add the sour cream, mayo, bleu cheese, mustard, and the seasoning and mix until creamy enough for your taste. Slice up the bacon to small pieces. Stir in the rest of the ingredients and fill up the eggs.

Nutrition: Calories: 217 kcal Fats: 16 g Carbs: 1 g
Protein: 6 g

Spinach Stuffed Chicken Breasts

Preparation Time: 25 minutes

Cooking Time: 15 minutes

Servings: 4

Ingredients:

- 1 ½ lbs. chicken breasts
- 4 ozs. cream cheese
- ¼ cup frozen spinach
- ½ cup mozzarella
- 4 oz. artichoke hearts
- ¼ cup Greek yogurt
- salt and pepper
- 2 tbsps. olive oil

Directions:

1. Pound the breasts about 1 inch thick. Cut each chicken down the middle, but don't cut through it. Make a pocket for the filling: season the chicken.
2. In a bowl, combine the Greek yogurt, mozzarella, cream cheese, artichoke, and spinach. Next, season it. Mix until well-combined.
3. Fill all breasts equally with your mixture.

4. In a skillet over medium heat, add the oil and place your chicken. Cover the skillet and cook for 5-6 mins, turning the heat up in the last 1-2 mins.

Nutrition: Calories: 288 kcal Fats: 18 g Carbs: 3 g Protein: 31 g

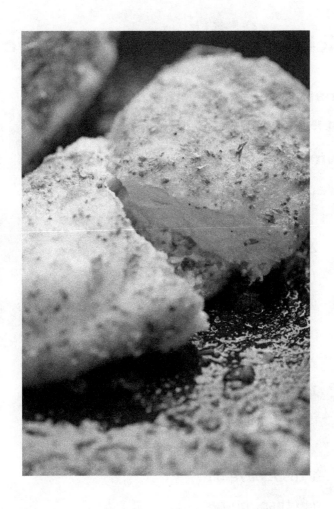

Chicken with Lemon and Garlic

Preparation Time: 5 minutes

Cooking Time: 20 minutes

Servings: 4

Ingredients:

- 4 boneless chicken thighs
- 2 garlic cloves minced
- Juice of 1 lemon
- ¼ tsp. smoked paprika, red chili flakes, garlic powder
- 2 tsps. Italian seasoning
- 1 tbsp. heavy cream
- fresh parsley
- ¼ small onion
- 1 tbsp. olive oil
- 1½ tbsp. butter
- salt and pepper

Directions:

1. Season your chicken with all spices.
2. In a skillet over medium heat, add the olive oil and cook for 5-6 mins on each side. Set aside on a plate.

3. Heat the skillet again and add in the butter. Stir in onion and garlic and add your lemon juice. Season them with everything left. After that, stir in your heavy cream. Once the sauce has thickened up, add the chicken back to the pot.

4. Serve it with lemon slices.

Nutrition: Calories: 279 kcal Fats: 15 g Carbs: 3 g Protein: 15 g

Chicken Pot Pie in a Slow Cooker

Preparation Time: 3 hours

Cooking Time: 35 minutes

Servings: 6

Ingredients:

- For the filling:
- 1 cup chicken broth
- ¾ cup heavy whipping cream
- 3 ½ oz. cooked chicken
- ½ cup mixed veggies
- ¼ onion
- 2 garlic cloves
- salt and pepper
- ¼ tsp. rosemary
- 1 tsp. poultry seasoning
- For the crust:
- 4 eggs
- 4 ½ tbsps. butter
- 1/3 cup coconut flour
- 1 1/3 cup shredded cheddar
- 2 tsps. full-fat sour cream
- ¼ tsp. baking powder

Directions:

1. Cook 1-1 ½ lbs. chicken in the slow cooker for 3 hours on high.
2. Preheat your oven to 400°F.
3. Sauté your onion, veggies, garlic cloves and season with 2 tbsp. butter in a skillet for 5-6 mins.
4. Add in the whipping cream, chicken broth, poultry, thyme, and rosemary.
5. Simmer them covered for 5 mins and don't forget to use a lot of liquid; otherwise, it will be really dry. Add the diced chicken, too.
6. Make the breading by mixing melted butter, salt, sour cream, and eggs before whisking them.
7. Add coconut flour and baking powder and stir until well-combined.
8. Stir in the cheddar cheese.
9. Bake in a 400°F oven for 15-20 mins.
10. Set oven to broil and move the pie to the top shelf. Broil for 2-4 mins to brown nicely.

Nutrition: Calories: 301 kcal Carbs: 5 g Protein: 15 g Fats: 24 g

Cheese Cauli Breadsticks

Preparation Time: 10 minutes

Cooking Time: 35 minutes

Servings: 6

Ingredients:

- 4 eggs
- 4 cups cauli
- 3 cups mozzarella cheese
- 4 cloves garlic
- 3 tsps. oregano
- salt and pepper

Directions:

1. Preheat your oven 425°F. Prepare one baking sheet with paper on it.
2. Chop your cauli to florets. Add them to a food processor and then pulse.
3. Microwave it for 10 mins and then let it cool afterward. In a large bowl, add in the cauli, eggs, 2 cups of cheese, oregano, garlic and season it, while mixing it.
4. Place the mixture on your sheet while forming your desired shape. Bake it for 20-25 mins.

Finally, top it with the rest of the cheese and bake for another 5 mins until golden and well melted.

Nutrition: Calories: 185 kcal Carbs: 4g Protein: 11 g Fats: 12 g

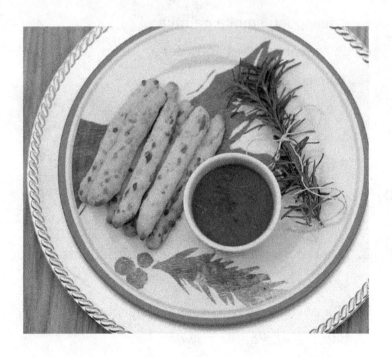

Baked Crispy Chicken

Preparation Time: 10 minutes

Cooking Time: 40 minutes

Servings: 12

Ingredients:

- 4 oz. pork rinds
- Salt and pepper to taste
- 1 teaspoon oregano
- 1 ½ teaspoons thyme
- 1 teaspoon smoke paprika
- ½ teaspoon garlic powder
- 12 chicken legs
- 2 oz. mayonnaise
- 1 egg
- 3 tablespoons Dijon mustard

Directions:

1. Preheat your oven to 400 degrees F.
2. Grind pork rinds until they've turned into powdery texture.
3. Mix pork rinds with salt, pepper, oregano, thyme, paprika and garlic powder.
4. Spread mixture on a plate.
5. In a bowl, mix the mayo, egg and mustard.

6. Dip each chicken leg first into the egg mixture then coat with the pork rind mixture.

7. Bake in the oven for 40 minutes.

Nutrition: Calories 359 Total Fat 16.3g Saturated Fat 4.7g Cholesterol 158mg Sodium 391mg Total Carbohydrate 1.6g Dietary Fiber 0.3g Total Sugars 0.4g Protein 49g Potassium 370mg

Italian Chicken

Preparation Time: 10 minutes

Cooking Time: 15 minutes

Servings: 4

Ingredients:

- 2 tablespoons olive oil
- 1 ½ lb. chicken breast meat, sliced thinly
- ½ cup chicken broth
- 1 cup heavy cream
- 1 teaspoon Italian seasoning
- ½ cup Parmesan cheese
- 1 teaspoon garlic powder
- 1 cup spinach, chopped
- ½ cup sun dried tomatoes

Directions:

- In a pan over medium heat, add olive oil.
- Cook chicken for 4 to 5 minutes per side.
- Transfer chicken on a plate.
- Stir in the broth, cream, Italian seasoning, and Parmesan cheese and garlic powder.
- Simmer until the sauce has thickened.
- Add the tomatoes and spinach.
- Cook until the spinach has wilted.

- Put the chicken back to the pan and serve.

Nutrition: Calories 535 Total Fat 29.4g Saturated Fat 11g Cholesterol 199mg Sodium 317mg Total Carbohydrate 6.1g Dietary Fiber 1g Total Sugars 0.4g Protein 60.3g Potassium 783mg

Chicken & Carrots

Preparation Time: 15 minutes

Cooking Time: 20 minutes

Servings: 4

Ingredients:

- 1 ½ lb. carrots, peeled and sliced
- 1 onion, sliced into quarters
- 1 head garlic, top sliced off
- 4 tablespoons olive oil, divided
- Salt and pepper to taste
- 1 tablespoon fresh rosemary, chopped
- 4 chicken thighs

Directions:

1. Preheat your oven to 425 degrees F.
2. Arrange the onion and carrots on a single layer on a baking pan.
3. Place the garlic in the middle of the tray.
4. Drizzle half of the olive oil over the vegetables.
5. Season with salt, pepper and rosemary.
6. Coat the chicken with the remaining oil.
7. Season with salt and pepper.
8. Bake in the oven for 20 minutes.

Nutrition: Calories 532 Total Fat 25.2g Saturated Fat 5.1g Cholesterol 130mg Sodium 250mg Total Carbohydrate 31.1g Dietary Fiber 5.8g Total Sugars 9.9g Protein 46.1g Potassium 1083mg

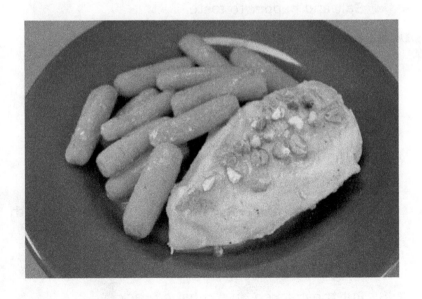

Lemon & Herb Chicken

Preparation Time: 20 minutes

Cooking Time: 60 minutes

Servings: 6

Ingredients:

- 1 whole chicken
- 4 tablespoons unsalted butter
- 3 lemons, sliced in half
- ½ bunch thyme
- ½ bunch rosemary
- Salt and pepper to taste

Directions:

1. Preheat your oven to 425 degrees F.
2. Cover the baking pan with foil.
3. Put a roasting rack on top.
4. Rub the chicken with butter.
5. Stuff the insides with lemon slices and herbs.
6. Season both inside and outside of chicken with salt and pepper.
7. Use twine to tie the chicken legs together.
8. Put the chicken on a roasting rack.
9. Roast for 40 minutes.

10. Reduce heat to 375 degrees F and roast until chicken is fully cooked.

11. Let chicken rest for 15 minutes before slicing and serving.

Nutrition: Calories 504 Total Fat 36.1g Saturated Fat 15g Cholesterol 180mgSodium 216mg

Total Carbohydrate 4.3g Dietary Fiber 1.8g Total Sugars 0.8g Protein 42.6g Potassium 65mg

Chicken & Avocado Salad

Preparation Time: 5 minutes

Cooking Time: 15 minutes

Servings: 4

Ingredients:

- Chicken
- ¼ cup water
- 2 boneless chicken thigh fillets
- 2 tablespoons olive oil
- Salt and pepper to taste
- 1 teaspoon sweet chili powder
- 1 teaspoon dried thyme
- 4 cloves garlic
- Salad
- 2 cups arugula
- 1 cup purslane leaves
- 1 cup basil leaves
- ½ cup fresh dill
- ½ cup cherry tomatoes, sliced in half
- 1 tablespoon olives
- 1 avocado, sliced
- 1 teaspoon sesame seeds
- ½ tablespoon olive oil

- 2 tablespoons avocado dressing

Directions:

1. Pour water into a skillet.
2. Cook chicken over medium low heat for 5 minutes.
3. Drizzle olive oil over the chicken
4. Season with the salt, pepper, thyme and chili powder.
5. Cook until golden, flipping several times to cook evenly.
6. Chop the chicken.
7. Arrange all the ingredients for the salad in a bowl.
8. Put the chicken on top of the salad.
9. Drizzle with the avocado dressing and olive oil.
10. Sprinkle sesame seeds on top.

Nutrition: Calories 517 Total Fat 38.6g Saturated Fat 6.4g Cholesterol 70mg Sodium 368mg
Total Carbohydrate 27.3g Dietary Fiber 9.9g Total Sugars 7.2g Protein 22g Potassium 1102mg

Chicken Bowl

Preparation Time: 10 minutes

Cooking Time: 20 minutes

Servings: 4

Ingredients:

- Salt and pepper to taste
- 2 teaspoons basil
- 2 teaspoon rosemary
- 2 teaspoons thyme
- 1 teaspoon paprika
- 2 lb. chicken breast meat, sliced into bite sized pieces
- 1 ½ cups broccoli florets
- 1 onion, chopped
- 1 cup tomatoes
- 1 zucchini, chopped
- 2 teaspoons garlic, minced
- 2 tablespoons olive oil
- 2 cups cauliflower rice

Directions:

1. Preheat your oven to 450 degrees F.
2. Cover your baking pan with foil. Set aside.
3. In a bowl, mix salt, pepper and spices.

4. Put the chicken and vegetables on a baking pan.

5. Sprinkle the spice mixture and garlic over the vegetables and chicken.

6. Drizzle olive oil on top.

7. Bake in the oven for 20 minutes.

8. Broil the chicken for 2 minutes.

9. Serve the chicken and vegetables in a bowl on top of cauliflower rice.

Nutrition: Calories 558 Total Fat 19.1g Saturated Fat 4.4g Cholesterol 206mg Sodium 260mg Total Carbohydrate 14.2g Dietary Fiber 3.3g Total Sugars 5.9g Protein 80.3g Potassium 1039mg

Chicken with Bacon & Ranch Sauce

Preparation Time: 10 minutes

Cooking Time: 20 minutes

Servings: 4

Ingredients:

- 4 chicken breasts
- 1 teaspoon paprika
- 1 teaspoon garlic powder
- 1 teaspoon onion powder
- 1 tablespoon avocado oil
- 6 oz. cream cheese
- 1 tablespoon ranch seasoning powder
- 1 cup cheddar, grated
- 10 slices bacon, cooked and crumbled
- 2 tablespoons green onions, chopped

Directions:

1. Preheat your oven to 375 degrees F.
2. Season the chicken with the paprika, garlic powder and onion powder.
3. Pour the oil in a pan over medium heat.
4. Cook the chicken in a pan over medium heat.

5. Cook for 4 minutes per side.

6. In a bowl, mix the cream cheese and ranch seasoning.

7. Spread the cream cheese mixture on top of the chicken.

8. Top with the cheese.

9. Bake in the oven for 10 minutes.

10. Top with the bacon and green onion before serving.

Nutrition: Calories 743 Total Fat 48g Saturated Fat 20.2g Cholesterol 235mg Sodium 1523mg

Total Carbohydrate 4.1g Dietary Fiber 0.5g Total Sugars 0.8g Protein 70.3g Potassium 738mg

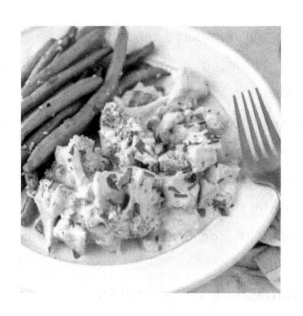

Creamy Chicken & Mushroom

Preparation Time: 10 minutes

Cooking Time: 20 minutes

Servings: 4

Ingredients:

- 1 lb. chicken tenderloin
- Salt and pepper to taste
- 2 tablespoons butter, divided
- 2 tablespoons olive oil, divided
- ½ lb. mushrooms, sliced
- 2 cloves garlic, crushed
- ¼ cup fresh parsley, chopped
- 2 tablespoons fresh thyme
- 1 cup chicken broth
- ½ cup heavy cream
- ¼ cup sour cream

Directions:

1. Season chicken with salt and pepper.
2. Add 1 tablespoon each of butter and olive oil in a pan.
3. Sear the chicken until brown on both sides.
4. Set aside.
5. Add the remaining oil and butter.

6. Cook the mushrooms until crispy.

7. Add the garlic, parsley and thyme.

8. Pour in the broth.

9. Stir in the cream and sour cream.

10.Simmer until the sauce has thickened.

11.Put the chicken back to the sauce.

Nutrition: Calories 383 Total Fat 23g Saturated Fat 10.1g Cholesterol 122mg Sodium 611mg Total Carbohydrate 4.7g Dietary Fiber 1.2g Total Sugars 1.3g Protein 42.1g Potassium 304mg

Mozzarella Chicken

Preparation Time: 10 minutes

Cooking Time: 20 minutes

Servings: 4

Ingredients:

- 4 chicken breasts (boneless, skinless)
- 1 tablespoon Italian seasoning, divided
- ½ teaspoon onion powder
- Salt and pepper to taste
- 1 teaspoon paprika
- 1 tablespoon olive oil
- 1 onion, chopped
- 4 cloves garlic, minced
- 1 fire roasted pepper, chopped
- 15 oz. tomato puree
- 2 tablespoons tomato paste
- ¾ cup mozzarella, shredded
- 1 tablespoons parsley, chopped

Directions:

1. Preheat your oven to 375 degrees F.
2. Season the chicken with 2 teaspoons Italian seasoning, onion powder, salt, pepper and paprika.

3. Pour the oil in a pan over medium heat.

4. Cook the chicken until brown on both sides.

5. Set aside.

6. Add the onion to the pan.

7. Cook for 3 minutes.

8. Add the garlic and pepper.

9. Cook for 1 minute.

10. Add the tomato puree and tomato paste. Mix well.

11. Stir in the remaining Italian sauce.

12. Simmer for 4 minutes.

13. Arrange the chicken on top of the sauce.

14. Add mozzarella on top.

15. Bake for 2 minutes.

16. Garnish with parsley before serving.

Nutrition: Calories 387 Total Fat 16.2g Saturated Fat 4.1g Cholesterol 130mg Sodium 193mg Total Carbohydrate 15.8g Dietary Fiber 3.3g Total Sugars 7.8g Protein 44.7g Potassium 963mg

Chicken Parmesan

Preparation Time: 20 minutes

Cooking Time: 8 minutes

Servings: 2

Ingredients:

- 2 chicken breast fillets
- 1 tablespoon heavy whipping cream
- 1 egg
- 1 ½ oz. pork rinds, crushed
- 1 oz. Parmesan cheese, grated
- Salt and pepper to taste
- ½ teaspoon garlic powder
- ½ teaspoon Italian seasoning
- 1 tablespoon ghee
- ½ cup tomato sauce
- ¼ cup mozzarella cheese, shredded

Directions:

1. Pound chicken fillet until flat.
2. In a bowl, mix the cream and egg.
3. Mix the pork rinds, Parmesan cheese, salt, pepper, garlic powder and Italian seasoning on another plate.
4. Dip the chicken fillet into the egg mixture.

5. Coat with the breading.

6. Add the ghee to a pan over medium heat.

7. Cook the chicken for 3 minutes per side.

8. Put the chicken to a baking pan.

9. Cover the top with tomato sauce and mozzarella cheese.

10. Broil for 2 minutes.

Nutrition: Calories 589 Total Fat 33.9g Saturated Fat 14.9g Cholesterol 282mg Sodium 1044mg Total Carbohydrate 5g Dietary Fiber 1g Total Sugars 3.1g Protein 65.3g Potassium 602mg

Spinach Frittata

Preparation Time: 10 minutes

Cooking Time: 35 minutes,

Servings: 4

Ingredients:

- 5 ounces of diced bacon
- 2 tablespoons of butter
- 8 ounces of spinach that's fresh
- 8 eggs
- A single cup of heavy whipping cream
- 5 ounces of shredded cheese

Directions:

1. Preheat your oven to 350 and grease a 9 by 9 baking dishes.
2. Fry your bacon on a heat medium until it is crispy.
3. Add your spinach and stir until it has wilted.
4. Remove pan from heat.
5. Place it to the side.
6. Whisk cream and eggs together and pour into the baking dish.
7. Add the spinach and bacon and pour the cheese on top.
8. Put in the middle of the oven.

9. Bake a half hour.

10. It should be set in the middle. The color on top should be golden brown.

Nutrition: Calories: 661g Fat: 59g Fiber: 1g Protein: 27 grams Carbs: 4 grams

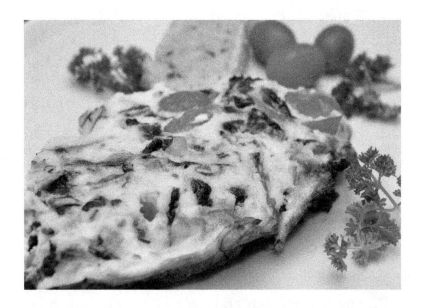

Muffins

Preparation Time: 15 minutes

Cooking time: 10mins

Servings: 12

Ingredients:

- 5 whisked medium eggs
- 2 cups of whole nuts

Directions:

1. Preheat oven to 350.
2. Grease a muffin tray (12 cups)
3. Process the nuts in a food processor.
4. Whisk eggs and nut flour, you made in a bowl.
5. Put in-tray.
6. Bake 25 minutes.
7. Stick should come out clean.
8. Let cool.

Nutrition: One muffin Calories: 117 Carbs: 4g Protein: 6g Fat: 10g

Halloumi Time

Preparation Time: 5 minutes

Cooking Time: 15 minutes

Servings: 2

Ingredients

- 3 ounces of halloumi cheese that has been diced
- 2 chopped scallions
- 4 ounces of diced bacon
- 2 tablespoons of olive oil
- 4 tablespoons of chopped fresh parsley
- 4 eggs
- Half a cup of pitted olives

Directions

1. In a frying pan on medium-high heat, heat the oil.
2. Fry the scallions, cheese, and bacon until they are nicely browned.
3. Get a bowl and whisk your eggs and parsley together.
4. Pour the egg mix into the pan over the bacon.
5. Lower heat.
6. Add olives.
7. Stir for 2 minutes.

Nutrition: Calories: 663g Protein: 28g Carbs: 4g
Fat: 59g

Hash Browns

Preparation Time: 20 minutes

Cooking Time: 10 minutes

Servings: 4

Ingredients:

- 3 eggs
- A pound of cauliflower
- Half a grated yellow onion
- 4 ounces of butter

Directions:

1. Rinse the cauliflower.
2. Trim it.
3. Grate it using a food processor.
4. Add it to a bowl.
5. Add everything and mix.
6. Set aside 10 minutes.
7. Melt a good amount of butter on medium heat.
8. You need a larger skillet.
9. Place the mix in the pan and flatten.
10. Fry for 5 minutes on each side.
11. Don't burn it.

Nutrition: Calories: 282 Carbs: 5g Protein: 7g Fat: 26g

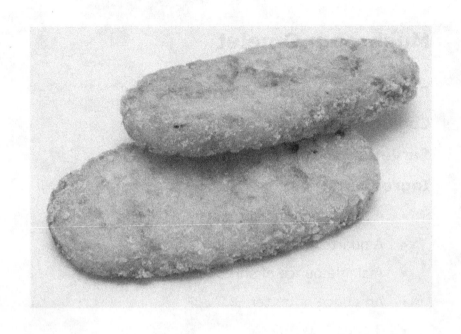

Mushroom Omelet

Preparation Time: 5minutes

Cooking Time: 10minutes

Servings: 1

Ingredients:

- 4 sliced large mushrooms
- A quarter chopped yellow onion
- A single ounce of shredded cheese
- An ounce of butter
- 3 eggs

Directions:

1. Crack the eggs and whisk them.
2. When smooth and frothy, they are good.
3. Melt butter over medium heat in a frying pan.
4. Add onions and mushrooms and stir until they become tender.
5. Pour the egg mix in. Surround the veggies.
6. When the omelet begins to get firm but is still a little raw on top, add cheese.
7. Carefully ease around the edges and fold in half.
8. When it's golden brown underneath (turning this color), remove and plate it.

Nutrition: Calories: 517g Protein: 26g Fat: 4g Carbs: 5g

Crab Melt

Preparation Time: 5 minutes

Cooking Time: 20 minutes

Servings: 4

Ingredients:

- 2 zucchinis
- A single tablespoon olive oil
- 3 ounces of stalks from celery
- 3/4 cup of mayo
- 12 ounces of crab meat
- A single red bell pepper
- 7 ounces of cheese (use shredded cheddar)
- A single tablespoon of Dijon mustard

Direction:

1. Preheat your oven to 450.
2. Slice your zucchini lengthwise. Go for about a half-inch thick.
3. Add salt.
4. Let it sit for 15 minutes.
5. Pat it dries with a paper towel.
6. Place your slices on a baking sheet.
7. The baking sheet needs to be lined with parchment paper.

8. Brush olive oil on each side.

9. Finely chop the vegetables.

10. Mix with the other ingredients.

11. Apply mix to zucchini.

12. Bake for 20 minutes. Your top will be golden brown.

Nutrition: Calories-742 Fat-65 grams Fiber-3 grams Carbs-7 grams Protein-30 grams

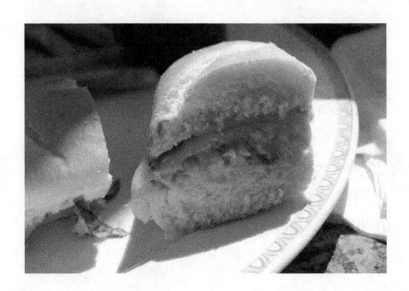

Poblano Peppers

Preparation Time: 5minutes

Cooking Time: 15minutes

Servings: 2

Ingredients

- A pound of grated cauliflower
- 3 ounces of butter
- 4 eggs
- 3 ounces of poblano peppers
- A single tablespoon of olive oil
- Half a cup of mayo

Directions:

1. Put your mayo in a bowl to the side.
2. Grate the cauliflower, including the stem.
3. Fry the cauliflower for 5 minutes in the butter.
4. Brush the oil on the peppers.
5. Fry them until you see the skin bubble a little.
6. Fry your eggs any way you like.
7. Serve with mayo.

Nutrition: Calories: 898 Fat: 87g Protein: 17g Carbs: 9g

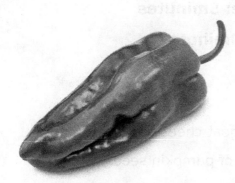

Salad with Butter

Preparation Time: 5minutes

Cooking Time: 10minutes

Servings: 2

Ingredients:

- 10 ounces of goat cheese
- A quarter cup of pumpkin seeds
- 2 ounces of butter
- Tablespoons of balsamic vinegar
- 3 ounces of spinach (use baby spinach)

Directions:

1. Preheat oven to 400.
2. Put goat cheese in a baking dish that is greased.
3. Bake 10 minutes.
4. Toast pumpkin seeds in a frying pan that is dry. The temperature should be fairly high. They need some color, and they should start to pop.
5. Lower heat.
6. Add butter and simmer till it smells nutty and is golden brown.
7. Add vinegar and boil 3 minutes.
8. Turn off heat.

9. Spread the spinach on your plate and top with cheese and sauce.

Nutrition: Calories: 824 Fat: 73g Protein: 37g Carbs: 3g

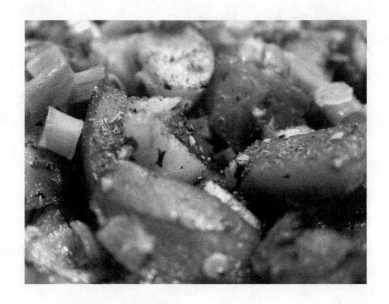

Tuna Casserole

Preparation Time 7minutes

Cooking Time 20minutes

Serving: 4

Ingredients:

- A single green bell pepper
- 5 ⅓ celery stalks
- 16 ounces of tuna in olive oil and drained
- A single yellow onion
- 2 ounces of butter
- A single cup of mayo
- 4 ounces of parmesan cheese freshly shredded
- A single teaspoon of chili flakes

Directions:

1. Preheat your oven to 400.
2. Chop all of the bell peppers, onions, and celery finely before frying it in butter in a frying pan. They should be slightly soft.
3. Mix mayo and tuna with the flakes and cheese.
4. This should be done in a greased baking dish.
5. Add the veggies.
6. Stir.
7. Bake 20 minutes.

8. It should be golden brown.

Nutrition: Calories: 953 Fat: 83g Protein: 43g
Carbs: 5g

Goat Cheese Frittata

Preparation Time: 15minutes

Cooking Time: 30minutes

Servings: 2

Ingredients:

- 4 ounces of goat cheese
- 5 ounces of mushrooms
- 3 ounces of fresh spinach
- 2 ounces of scallions
- 2 ounces of butter
- Half a dozen eggs

Directions:

1. Preheat your oven to 350.
2. Crack the eggs and whisk before crumbling cheese in the mix.
3. Cut mushrooms into wedge shapes.
4. Chop up the scallions.
5. Melt the butter in a skillet that is oven proof and cook scallions and mushrooms over medium heat for 10 minutes. They will be golden brown (or should be).
6. Add spinach and sauté two minutes.
7. Pour egg mixture into the skillet.

8. Place in the oven uncovered and bake 20 minutes.

9. It should be golden brown in the center.

Nutrition: Calories: 774 Fat: 67g Carbs: 6g Protein: 35g

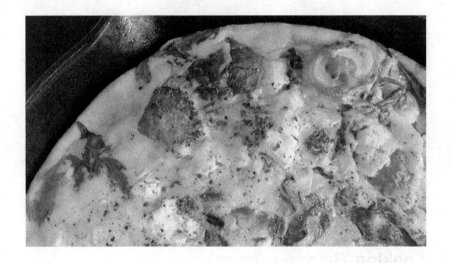

POULTRY

Pancakes

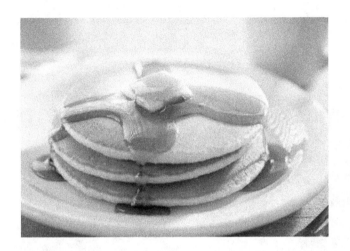

Preparation Time: 5 minutes

Cooking Time: 6 minutes

Servings: 2

Ingredients

- ¼ cup almond flour
- 1 ½ tbsp. unsalted butter
- 2 oz. cream cheese, softened
- 2 eggs

Directions:

1. Take a bowl, crack eggs in it, whisk well until fluffy, and then whisk in flour and cream cheese until well combined.
2. Take a skillet pan, place it over medium heat, add butter and when it melts, drop pancake batter in four sections, spread it evenly, and cook for 2 minutes per side until brown.
3. Serve.

Nutrition: 166.8 Calories; 15 g Fats; 5.8 g Protein; 1.8 g Net Carb; 0.8 g Fiber;

Cheese Roll-Ups

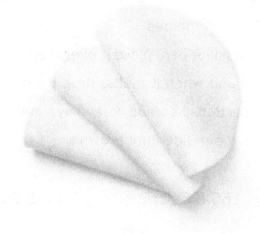

Preparation Time: 5 minutes

Cooking Time: 0 minutes

Servings: 2

Ingredients

- 2 oz. mozzarella cheese, sliced, full-fat
- 1-ounce butter, unsalted

Directions:

1. Cut cheese into slices and then cut butter into thin slices.
2. Top each cheese slice with a slice of butter, roll it and then serve.

Nutrition: 166 Calories; 15 g Fats; 6.5 g Protein; 2 g Net Carb; 0 g Fiber;

Scrambled Eggs with Spinach and Cheese

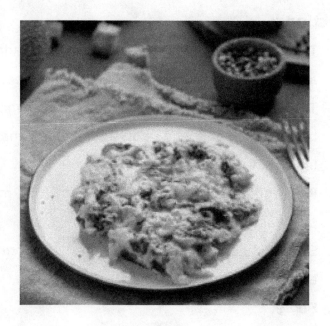

Preparation Time: 5 minutes

Cooking Time: 5 minutes

Servings: 2

Ingredients

- 2 oz. spinach
- 2 eggs
- 1 tbsp. coconut oil
- 2 tbsp. grated mozzarella cheese, full-fat
- Seasoning:

- ¼ tsp salt
- 1/8 tsp ground black pepper
- 1/8 tsp red pepper flakes

Directions:

1. Take a medium bowl, crack eggs in it, add salt and black pepper and whisk until combined.
2. Take a medium skillet pan, place it over medium heat, add oil and when hot, add spinach and cook for 1 minute until leaves wilt.
3. Pour eggs over spinach, stir and cook for 1 minute until just set.
4. Stir in cheese, then remove the pan from heat and sprinkle red pepper flakes on top.
5. Serve.

Nutrition: 171 Calories; 14 g Fats; 9.2 g Protein; 1.1 g Net Carb; 1.7 g Fiber;

Egg Wraps

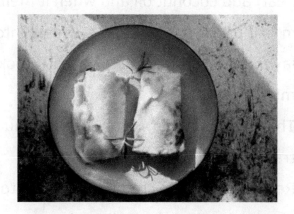

Preparation Time: 5 minutes

Cooking Time: 5 minutes

Servings: 2

Ingredients

- 2 eggs
- 1 tbsp. coconut oil
- Seasoning:
- ¼ tsp salt
- 1/8 tsp ground black pepper

Directions:

Take a medium bowl, crack eggs in it, add salt and black pepper, and then whisk until blended.

Take a frying pan, place it over medium-low heat, add coconut oil and when it melts, pour in half of the egg, spread it evenly into a thin layer by rotating the pan and cook for 2 minutes.

Then flip the pan, cook for 1 minute, and transfer to a plate.

Repeat with the remaining egg to make another wrap, then roll each egg wrap and serve.

Nutrition: 68 Calories; 4.7 g Fats; 5.5 g Protein; 0.5 g Net Carb; 0 g Fiber;

Chaffles with Poached Eggs

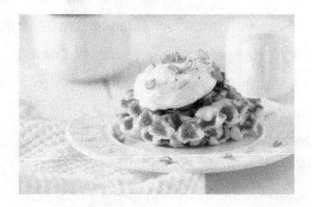

Preparation Time: 5 minutes

Cooking Time: 10 minutes

Servings: 2

Ingredients

- 2 tsp coconut flour
- ½ cup shredded cheddar cheese, full-fat
- 3 eggs
- Seasoning:
- ¼ tsp salt
- 1/8 tsp ground black pepper

Directions:

1. Switch on a mini waffle maker and let it preheat for 5 minutes.

2. Meanwhile, take a medium bowl, place all the ingredients in it, reserving 2 eggs and then mix by using an immersion blender until smooth.

3. Ladle the batter evenly into the waffle maker, shut with lid, and let it cook for 3 to 4 minutes until firm and golden brown.

4. Meanwhile, prepare poached eggs, and for this, take a medium bowl half full with water, place it over medium heat and bring it to a boil.

5. Then crack an egg in a ramekin, carefully pour it into the boiling water and cook for 3 minutes.

6. Transfer egg to a plate lined with paper towels by using a slotted spoon and repeat with the other egg.

7. Top chaffles with poached eggs, season with salt and black pepper, and then serve.

Nutrition: 265 Calories; 18.5 g Fats; 17.6 g Protein; 3.4 g Net Carb; 6 g Fiber;

Chaffle with Scrambled Eggs

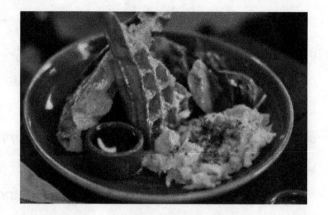

Preparation Time: 5 minutes

Cooking Time: 10 minutes

Servings: 2

Ingredients

- 2 tsp coconut flour
- ½ cup shredded cheddar cheese, full-fat
- 3 eggs
- 1-ounce butter, unsalted
- Seasoning:
- ¼ tsp salt
- 1/8 tsp ground black pepper
- 1/8 tsp dried oregano

Directions:

1. Switch on a mini waffle maker and let it preheat for 5 minutes.
2. Meanwhile, take a medium bowl, place all the ingredients in it, reserving 2 eggs and then mix by using an immersion blender until smooth.
3. Ladle the batter evenly into the waffle maker, shut with lid, and let it cook for 3 to 4 minutes until firm and golden brown.
4. Meanwhile, prepare scrambled eggs and for this, take a medium bowl, crack the eggs in it and whisk them with a fork until frothy, and then season with salt and black pepper.
5. Take a medium skillet pan, place it over medium heat, add butter and when it melts, pour in eggs and cook for 2 minutes until creamy, stirring continuously.
6. Top chaffles with scrambled eggs, sprinkle with oregano, and then serve.

Nutrition: 265 Calories; 18.5 g Fats; 17.6 g Protein; 3.4 g Net Carb; 6 g Fiber;

Sheet Pan Eggs with Mushrooms and Spinach

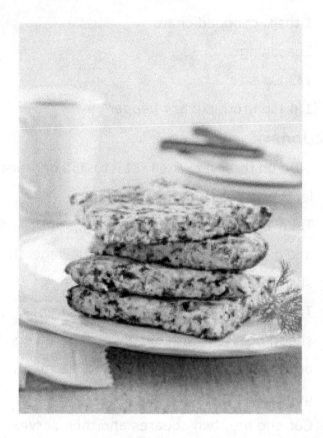

Preparation Time: 5 minutes

Cooking Time: 12 minutes

Servings: 2

Ingredients

- 2 eggs

- 1 tsp chopped jalapeno pepper
- 1 tbsp. chopped mushrooms
- 1 tbsp. chopped spinach
- 1 tbsp. chopped chard
- Seasoning:
- 1/3 tsp salt
- 1/4 tsp ground black pepper

Directions:

1. Turn on the oven, then set it to 350 degrees F and let it preheat.
2. Take a medium bowl, crack eggs in it, add salt and black pepper, then add all the vegetables and stir until combined.
3. Take a medium sheet ball or rimmed baking sheet, grease it with oil, pour prepared egg batter on it, and then bake for 10 to 12 minutes until done.
4. Cut egg into two squares and then serve.

Nutrition: 165 Calories; 10.7 g Fats; 14 g Protein; 1.5 g Net Carb; 0.5 g Fiber;

No Bread Breakfast Sandwich

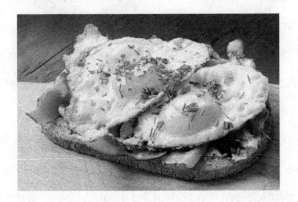

Preparation Time: 10 minutes

Cooking Time: 15 minutes

Servings: 2

Ingredients

- 2 slices of ham
- 4 eggs
- 1 tsp tabasco sauce
- 3 tbsp. butter, unsalted
- 2 tsp grated mozzarella cheese
- Seasoning:
- ¼ tsp salt
- 1/8 tsp ground black pepper

Directions:

1. Take a frying pan, place it over medium heat, add butter and when it melt, crack an egg in it and fry for 2 to 3 minutes until cooked to desired level.

2. Transfer fried egg to a plate, fry remaining eggs in the same manner and when done, season eggs with salt and black pepper.

3. Prepare the sandwich and for this, use a fried egg as a base for sandwich, then top with a ham slice, sprinkle with a tsp of ham and cover with another fried egg.

4. Place egg into the pan, return it over low heat and let it cook until cheese melts.

5. Prepare another sandwich in the same manner and then serve.

Nutrition: 180 Calories; 15 g Fats; 10 g Protein; 1 g Net Carb; 0 g Fiber;

Scrambled Eggs with Basil and Butter

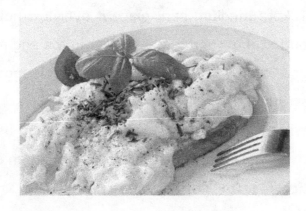

Preparation Time: 5 minutes

Cooking Time: 5 minutes

Servings: 2

Ingredients

- 1 tbsp. chopped basil leaves
- 2 tbsp. butter, unsalted
- 2 tbsp. grated cheddar cheese
- 2 eggs
- 2 tbsp. whipping cream
- Seasoning:
- 1/8 tsp salt
- 1/8 tsp ground black pepper

Directions:

1. Take a medium bowl, crack eggs in it, add salt, black pepper, cheese and cream and whisk until combined.

2. Take a medium pan, place it over low heat, add butter and when it melts, pour in the egg mixture and cook for 2 to 3 minutes until eggs have scrambled to the desired level.

3. When done, distribute scrambled eggs between two plates, top with basil leaves and then serve.

Nutrition: 320 Calories; 29 g Fats; 13 g Protein; 1.5 g Net Carb; 0 g Fiber;

Bacon, and Eggs

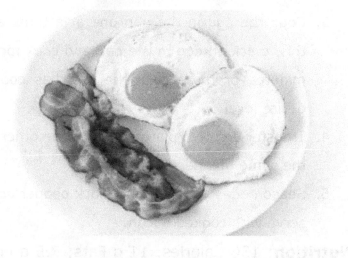

Preparation Time: 5 minutes

Cooking Time: 10 minutes

Servings: 2

Ingredients

- 2 eggs
- 4 slices of turkey bacon
- ¼ tsp salt
- ¼ tsp ground black pepper

Directions:

1. Take a skillet pan, place it over medium heat, add bacon slices in it and cook for 5 minutes until crispy.

2. Transfer bacon slices to a plate and set aside until required, reserving the fat in the pan.

3. Cook the egg in the pan one at a time, and for this, crack an egg in the pan and cook for 2 to 3 minutes or more until the egg has cooked to desire level.

4. Transfer egg to a plate and cook the other egg in the same manner.

5. Season eggs with salt and black pepper and then serve with cooked bacon.

Nutrition: 136 Calories; 11 g Fats; 7.5 g Protein; 1 g Net Carb; 0 g Fiber

Boiled Eggs

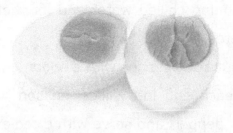

Preparation Time: 5 minutes

Cooking Time: 10 minutes

Servings: 2

Ingredients

- 2 eggs
- ½ of a medium avocado
- Seasoning:
- ¼ tsp salt
- ¼ tsp ground black pepper

Directions:

1. Place a medium pot over medium heat, fill it half full with water and bring it to boil.
2. Then carefully place the eggs in the boiling water and boil the eggs for 5 minutes until soft-boiled,

8 minutes for medium-boiled, and 10 minutes for hard-boiled.

3. When eggs have boiled, transfer them to a bowl containing chilled water and let them rest for 5 minutes.

4. Then crack the eggs with a spoon and peel them.

5. Cut each egg into slices, season with salt and black pepper, and serve with diced avocado.

Nutrition: 112 Calories; 9.5 g Fats; 5.5 g Protein; 1 g Net Carb; 0 g Fiber;

Spicy Cheese Chicken Soup

Preparation Time: 15 MINUTES

Cooking Time: 40 MINUTES

Servings: 4

Ingredients

- ½ cup salsa enchilada verde
- 2 cups chicken, cooked and shredded
- 2 cups chicken or bone broth
- 1 cup cheddar cheese, shredded
- 4 ounces cream cheese
- ½ tsp chili powder
- ½ tsp cumin, ground
- ½ tsp fresh cilantro, chopped
- Salt and black pepper to taste

Directions

1. Combine the cream cheese, salsa verde, and broth in a food processor.
2. Pulse until smooth. Transfer the mixture to a pot and place over medium heat.
3. Cook until hot, but do not bring to a boil.
4. Add chicken, chili powder, and cumin, and cook for about 3-5 minutes, or until it is heated

through. Stir in Cheddar cheese. Season with salt and pepper to taste.

5. Serve hot in individual bowls sprinkled with fresh cilantro.

Nutrition Calories 346, Net Carbs 3g, Fat 23g, Protein 25g

Cheese & Spinach Stuffed Chicken

Preparation Time: 50 MINUTES

Cooking Time: 40 MINUTES

Servings: 4

Ingredients

- 4 chicken breasts, boneless and skinless
- ½ cup mozzarella cheese
- 1 ½ cups Parmesan cheese, shredded
- 6 ounces cream cheese
- 2 cups spinach, chopped
- A pinch of nutmeg
- ½ tsp garlic, minced
- <u>Breading</u>
- 2 eggs, beaten
- 1/3 cup almond flour
- 2 tbsp. olive oil
- ½ tsp parsley
- 1/3 cup Parmesan cheese
- A pinch of onion powder

Directions

1. Pound the chicken until it doubles in size. Mix cream cheese, spinach, mozzarella cheese, nutmeg, and salt, pepper, and Parmesan cheese

in a bowl. Divide the mixture between the chicken breasts and spread it out evenly. Wrap the chicken in a plastic wrap. Refrigerate for 15 minutes.

2. Preheat the oven to 370 F.
3. Beat the eggs and set aside. Combine all of the other breading ingredients in a bowl. Dip the chicken in eggs first, then in the breading mixture.
4. Warm the olive oil in a pan over medium heat. Cook the chicken in the pan until browned, about 5-6 minutes. Place on a lined baking sheet, and bake for 20 minutes. Serve.

Nutrition Calories 491, Net Carbs 3.5g, Fat 36g, Protein 38g

Chicken & Spinach Gratin

Preparation Time: 45 MINUTES

Cooking Time: 40 MINUTES

Servings: 6

Ingredients

- 6 chicken breasts, skinless and boneless
- 1 tsp mixed spice seasoning
- Pink salt and black pepper to season
- 2 loose cups baby spinach
- 3 tsp olive oil
- 4 oz. cream cheese, cubed
- 1 ¼ cups mozzarella cheese, shredded
- 4 tbsp. water

Directions

1. Preheat oven to 375 F.
2. Season chicken with spice mix, salt, and black pepper. Pat with your hands to have the seasoning stick on the chicken.
3. Put in the casserole dish and layer spinach over the chicken.
4. Mix the oil with cream cheese, mozzarella, salt, and black pepper and stir in water a tablespoon at a time.

5. Pour the mixture over the chicken and cover the pot with aluminum foil.

6. Bake for 20 minutes, remove foil and continue cooking for 15 minutes until a beautiful golden brown color is formed on top.

7. Take out and allow sitting for 5 minutes. Serve warm with braised asparagus.

Nutrition Calories 340, Net Carbs 1g, Fat 30.2g, Protein 15g

Weekend Chicken with Grapefruit & Lemon

Preparation Time: 30 MINUTES

Cooking Time: 40 MINUTES

Servings: 4

Ingredients

- 1 cup omission IPA
- A pinch of garlic powder
- 1 tsp grapefruit zest
- 3 tbsp. lemon juice
- ½ tsp coriander, ground
- 1 tbsp. fish sauce
- 2 tbsp. butter
- ¼ tsp xanthan gum
- 3 tbsp. swerve sweetener
- 20 chicken wing pieces
- Salt and black pepper to taste

Directions

1. Combine lemon juice and zest, fish sauce, coriander, omission IPA, sweetener, and garlic powder in a saucepan.

2. Bring to a boil, cover, lower the heat, and let simmer for 10 minutes.

3. Stir in the butter and xanthan gum. Set aside. Season the wings with some salt and pepper.

4. Preheat the grill and cook for 5 minutes per side.

5. Serve topped with the sauce.

Nutrition Calories 365, Net Carbs 4g, Fat 25g, Protein 21g

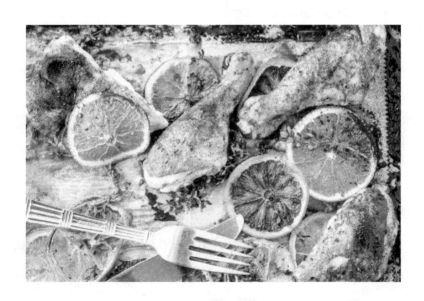

Bacon-Wrapped Chicken with Grilled Asparagus

Preparation Time: 50 MINUTES

Cooking Time: 40 MINUTES

Servings: 4

Ingredients

- 2 tbsp. fresh lemon juice
- 6 chicken breasts
- 8 bacon slices
- 1 tbsp. olive oil
- 1 lb. asparagus spears
- 3 tbsp. olive oil
- Salt and black pepper to taste
- Manchego cheese for topping

Directions

1. Preheat the oven to 400 F.

2. Season chicken breasts with salt and black pepper, and wrap 2 bacon slices around each chicken breast. Arrange on a baking sheet that is lined with parchment paper, drizzle with oil, and bake for 25-30 minutes until bacon is brown and crispy.

3. Preheat the grill.

4. Brush the asparagus spears with olive oil and season with salt. Grill turning frequently until slightly charred, 5-10 minutes.

5. Remove to a plate and drizzle with lemon juice. Grate over Manchego cheese so that it melts a little on contact with the hot asparagus and forms a cheesy dressing.

Nutrition Calories 468, Net Carbs 2g, Fat 38g, Protein 26g

Bok Choy Caesar Salad with Chicken

PREPARATION TIME: 1 HOUR AND 20 MINUTES

COOKING TIME: 40 MINUTES

SERVINGS: 4

Ingredients

- Chicken
- 4 chicken thighs, boneless and skinless
- ¼ cup lemon juice
- 2 garlic cloves, minced
- 2 tbsp. olive oil
- Salad
- ½ cup caesar salad dressing, sugar-free
- 2 tbsp. olive oil
- 12 bok choy leaves
- 3 Parmesan cheese crisps
- Parmesan cheese, grated or garnishing

Directions

1. Combine the chicken ingredients in a Ziploc bag. Seal the bag, shake to combine, and refrigerate for 1 hour.

2. Preheat the grill to medium heat, and grill the chicken about 4 minutes per side.

3. Cut bok choy leaves lengthwise, and brush it with oil. Grill for about 3 minutes. Place on a serving platter. Top with the chicken, and drizzle the dressing over. Sprinkle with Parmesan cheese and finish with Parmesan crisps to serve.

Nutrition Calories 529, Net Carbs 5g, Fat 39g, Protein 33g

Turkey Patties with Cucumber Salsa

Preparation Time: 30 MINUTES

Cooking Time: 40 MINUTES

Servings: 4

Ingredients

- 2 spring onions, thinly sliced
- 1 pound turkey, ground
- 1 egg
- 2 garlic cloves, minced
- 1 tbsp. herbs, chopped
- 1 small chili pepper, deseeded and diced
- 2 tbsp. ghee
- Cucumber Salsa:
- 1 tbsp. apple cider vinegar
- 1 tbsp. dill, chopped
- 1 garlic clove, minced
- 2 cucumbers, grated
- 1 cup sour cream
- 1 jalapeño pepper, minced
- 2 tbsp. olive oil

Directions

1. Place all of the turkey ingredients, except the ghee, in a bowl. Mix to combine. Make patties out of the mixture.
2. Melt ghee in a skillet over medium heat. Cook the patties for 3 minutes per side.
3. Place all of the salsa ingredients in a bowl and mix to combine. Serve the patties topped with salsa.

Nutrition Calories 475, Net Carbs 5g, Fat 38g, Protein 26g

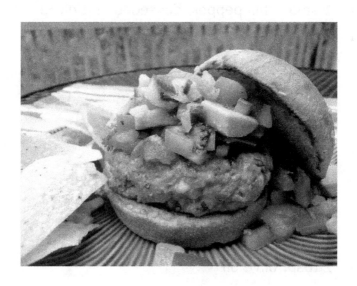

Chili Chicken Kabobs with Tahini Dressing

Preparation Time: 20 MINUTES+ 2 HOURS REFRIGERATION

Cooking Time: 10 MINUTES

Servings: 6

Ingredients

- 3 tbsp. soy sauce
- 1 tbsp. ginger-garlic paste
- 2 tbsp. swerve brown sugar
- 2 tbsp. olive oil
- 3 chicken breasts, cut into bite-sized cubes
- ½ cup tahini
- ½ tsp garlic powder
- Salt and chili pepper to taste

Directions

1. In a bowl, whisk soy sauce, ginger-garlic paste, swerve brown sugar, chili pepper, and olive oil. Put the chicken in a zipper bag, pour the marinade over, seal, and shake for an even coat. Marinate in the fridge for 2 hours.

2. Preheat a grill to 400 F and thread the chicken on skewers. Cook for 10 minutes in total with three to four turnings to be golden brown. Plate them.

3. Mix the tahini, garlic powder, salt, and ¼ cup of warm water in a bowl. Serve the chicken skewers and tahini dressing with cauliflower fried rice.

Nutrition Calories 225, Net Carbs 2g, Fat 17.4g, Protein 15g

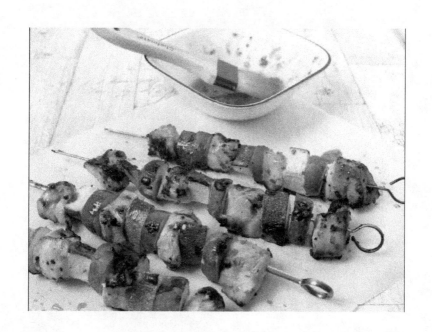

CONCLUSION

The things to watch out for when coming off keto are weight gain, bloating, more energy, and feeling hungry. The weight gain is nothing to freak out over; perhaps, you might not even gain any. It all depends on your diet, how your body processes carbs, and, of course, water weight. The length of your keto diet is a significant factor in how much weight you have lost, which is caused by the reduction of carbs. The bloating will occur because of the reintroduction of fibrous foods and your body getting used to digesting them again. The bloating van lasts for a few days to a few weeks. You will feel like you have more energy because carbs break down into glucose, which is the body's primary source of fuel. You may also notice better brain function and the ability to work out more.

Whether you have met your weight loss goals, your life changes, or you simply want to eat whatever you want again. You cannot just suddenly start consuming carbs again for it will shock your system. Have an idea of what you want to allow back into your consumption slowly. Be familiar with portion sizes and stick to that amount of carbs for the first few times you eat post-keto.

Start with non-processed carbs like whole grain, beans, and fruits. Start slow and see how your body responds before resolving to add carbs one meal at a time.

The ketogenic diet is the ultimate tool you can use to plan your future. Can you picture being more involved, more productive and efficient, and more relaxed and energetic? That future is possible for you, and it does not have to be a complicated process to achieve that vision. You can choose right now to be healthier and slimmer and more fulfilled tomorrow. It is possible with the ketogenic diet.

It does not just improve your physical health but your mental and emotional health as well. This diet improves your health holistically. Do not give up now as there will be quite a few days where you may think to yourself, "Why am I doing this?" and to answer that, simply focus on the goals you wish to achieve.

A good diet enriched with all the proper nutrients is our best shot of achieving an active metabolism and efficient lifestyle. A lot of people think that the Keto diet is simply for people who are interested in losing weight. You will find that it is quite the opposite. There are intense keto diets where only 5 percent of the diet comes from carbs, 20 percent is from protein, and 75 percent is from fat. But even a modified version of this which involves consciously choosing foods low in carbohydrate and high in healthy fats is good enough.

Thanks for reading this book. I hope it has provided you with enough insight to get you going. Don't put off getting started. The sooner you begin this diet, the sooner you'll start to notice an improvement in your health and well-being.

CPSIA information can be obtained
at www.ICGtesting.com
Printed in the USA
BVHW041750080421
604549BV00012B/262

9 781801 834780